Anti-Inflammatory Diet Cookbook

50 Healthy and Delicious Recipes to Reduce Inflammation and Boost Autoimmune System

Gena Pemberton

Table of Contents

Introduction

An anti-inflammatory diet should contain a recommended daily intake of 2,000 – 3,000 calories, 67 grams of fat and 2,300 mg of sodium. Fifty percent (50%) of those calories should come from carbohydrates, twenty percent (20%) should

come from protein and the remaining thirty percent (30%) should come from fat.

You can get carbohydrate-rich foods from eating whole-wheat grains, sweet potatoes, squash, bulgur wheat, beans and brown rice.

On the other hand, your intake of fat should come from most types of fish and any foods cooked in extra-virgin olive oil or organic canola oil. You can get protein from soybeans and other whole-soy products.

This diet prohibits fast food or processed food in any part of the meal. This also means a restriction on pork, beef, butter, cream and margarine. The antiinflammatory diet should also contain less processed sugar for diabetics and low cholesterol (though Omega-3, which is found in a variety of fish, is a good cholesterol) for people with heart problems.

Benefits of an anti-inflammatory diet

One of the benefits of an anti-inflammatory diet is that it uses fresh foods with phytonutrients that prevent degenerative ailments from occurring. The diet plan also produces cardiovascular benefits; thanks to the inclusion of the Omega-3

fatty acids. These fatty acids aid in preventing complications in the heart and reducing the levels of "bad" cholesterol and blood pressure.

Another benefit of the anti-inflammatory diet is that it is diabetic friendly. As

this diet restricts processed sugar and sugar-loaded meals and snacks, it works

perfectly for patients who are suffering diabetes. While the diet does not

substantially reduce weight, it decreases a patient's likelihood of suffering from

obesity. This is due to the inclusion of natural fruits and vegetables, and the

restriction of meat and other processed foods.

1. <u>Ginger Apple Muffins</u>

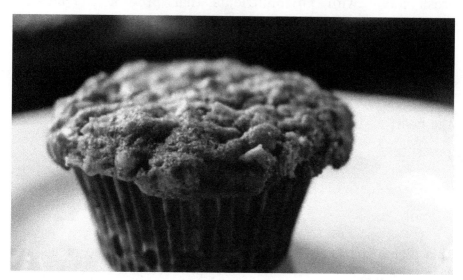

Ingredients:

- All-purpose flour (2 cups)
- Sugar or sugar-free sweeteners (2/3 cup)
- Baking powder (1 tbsp.)
- Salt (1/2 tsp.)
- Ground cinnamon (1 tsp.)
- Ground ginger (1 tsp.)
- Unsweetened almond milk (3/4 cup)
- Shredded apple (1 cup)
- Mashed ripe banana (1/2 cup)
- Apple cider vinegar (1 tbsp.)

Procedure:

1. Pre-heat the oven to 400'F.

2. Lightly grease the molds in a muffin pan, or use parchment paper to line up the molds.

3. Whisk together the flour, sugar, baking powder, salt, cinnamon and ginger in a mixing bowl until you form a smooth batter without any lumps.

4. In another mixing bowl, mix the almond milk, shredded apples, mashed banana and apple cider vinegar until the mixture is fully combined. Add the flour mixture and stir until the batter incorporates the milk mixture.

5. Fill the batter into the muffin molds, until the molds are 2/3 full.

6. Bake the muffins into the oven at 400'F for 15 – 20 minutes. When you insert a toothpick into a muffin and it comes clean, they are ready.

7. The ginger apple muffins yield 12 servings, with each muffin at approximately 170 calories. It has 0.6 mg fat, zero cholesterol, and 234 mg sodium.

2. <u>Spinach and Mushroom Frittatas</u>

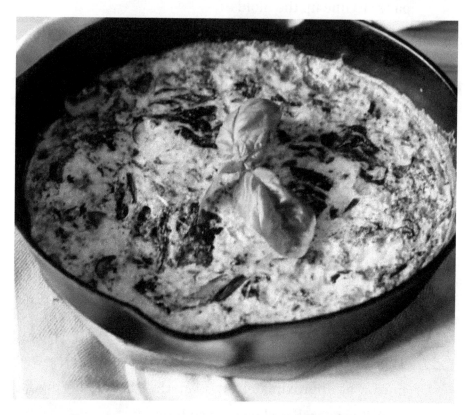

Ingredients:

- Sliced button mushrooms (1 lb.)
- Chopped large onion (1 pc.)
- Chopped garlic (1 tbsp.)
- Spinach (1 lb.)
- Water (1/4 cup)
- Egg whites (6 pcs.)
- Eggs (4 pcs.)
- Firm tofu (6 oz.)

- Ground turmeric (1/2 tsp.)
- Kosher salt (1/2 tsp.)
- Cracked or powdered black pepper (1/2 tsp.)

Procedure:

1. Pre-heat the oven to 350'F.
2. In a non-stick skillet or sauté pan, sauté the button mushrooms over medium to high heat. Add chopped onions and keep sautéing for 3 minutes or until the onions are tender.
3. Add water. Then add spinach to the skillet or pan and cook for 2 minutes with the lid on, or until the spinach wilts. Cook again until all the water is dispersed.
4. Set aside.
5. Puree, eggs, turmeric, salt, pepper, tofu and egg whites in a blender at medium or high speed until the mixture is smooth.
6. Gently pour the egg mixture into the spinach.
7. Bake the sauté pan into the oven for 25 – 30 minutes at 350'F. Once it's done, take the pan out, invert the frittata onto a plate and leave it for 10 minutes. Once it's done, cut the frittata into wedges and they're ready to be served.
8. The frittatas yield 6 – 8 servings. Each serving has 130 g fat, 123mg cholesterol and 362mg sodium.

3. Gluten-Free Strawberry Crepes

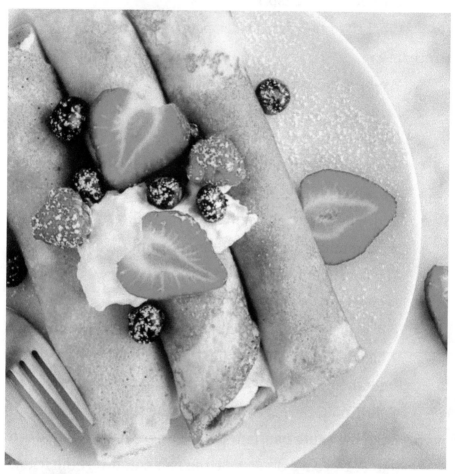

Ingredients:

- Sliced strawberries (6 cups)
- Sugar or honey (2 tbsp.)
- Large eggs (4 pcs.)
- Unsweetened almond milk (1 cup)
- Olive oil (2 tbsp.)
- Vanilla extract (1 tsp.)

- Light brown sugar (1 tsp.)
- Salt (1 tsp.)
- Gluten-free flour baking mix (3/4 cup)

Directions:

1. Mix strawberries and sugar until the strawberries are coated. Let it stand for 30 minutes at room temperature.

2. Put the eggs, almond milk, olive oil, vanilla extract, brown sugar and salt into a mixing bowl, then whisk it all together until all the ingredients are combined.

3. Add the gluten-free four and mix it until the batter is smooth and creamy.

4. Heat a non-stick skillet or crepe pan in a stove or oven on medium heat. Add ¼ cup of batter into the skillet and coat it evenly. Cook it for around 45 seconds or until the crepe starts to turn brown.

5. Flip the crepe over and cook the other side for 10 seconds then transfer it to a serving plate.

6. Take out ½ cup of the sugared strawberries with a spoon then put it on top of the crepe. Carefully fold the crepe as you cover the strawberries, in order to form a half-circle.

7. Drizzle the crepe with any syrup or juice then serve.

8. You will need to serve two strawberry crepes to make one serving. Each serving has 220 calories, 9.7g fat, 123 mg cholesterol and 130 mg sodium.

4. <u>Cherry Quinoa Porridge</u>

Ingredients:

- Water (1 cup)
- Dry quinoa (1/2 cup)
- Dried unsweetened cherries (1/2 cup)
- Vanilla extract (1/2 tsp.)
- Ground cinnamon (1/4 tsp.)
- Honey (1 tsp.)

Directions:

1. Stir together water, quinoa, cherries, vanilla extract and cinnamon in a medium-sized saucepan. Bring it to a boil over medium or high heat.

2. Simmer with the lid covering the saucepan for 15 minutes. The quinoa is ready when all the water has been absorbed and the porridge is tender.

3. Drizzle with honey then serve.

5. Raspberry Green Tea Smoothie

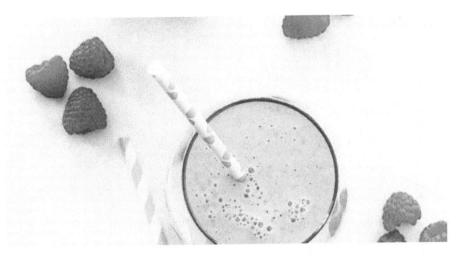

Ingredients:

- Chilled green tea (1 ½ cups)
- Frozen unsweetened raspberries (2 cups)
- Banana (1 pc.)
- Honey (1 tbsp.)
- Protein powder (1/4 cup)

Procedure:

1. Add all the ingredients into a blender.

2. Puree the ingredients until the mixture is very smooth and creamy.

3. Pour the puree into a tall glass and serve.

6. __Buckwheat and Quinoa Granola__

Ingredients:

- Honey (3 tbsp.)
- Liquid coconut oil (3 tbsp.)
- Vanilla extract (1 tsp.)
- Ground cinnamon (1/4 tsp.)
- Ground ginger (1/4 tsp.)
- Buckwheat oats (1 cup)
- Cooked quinoa (1 cup)
- Regular oats (1/2 cup)
- Dried unsweetened cranberries (1/2 cup)

Directions:

1. Line a baking sheet with parchment paper or silicon baking mat, or lightly

grease a sheet with olive oil. Preheat the oven to 325'F.

2. Stir together coconut oil, vanilla extract, honey, ginger and cinnamon into

a small mixing bowl.

3. In a separate large mixing bowl, mix the buckwheat, quinoa and oats

together.

4. Add the honey mixture and stir thoroughly until all the ingredients are

fully combined.

5. Spread the mixture evenly in a pan and bake at 325'F for 40 – 45 minutes or until it begins to brown.

6. Remove the pan and add the cranberries. Stir it well then place the pan on a cooling rack for it to cool completely.

7. Store the granola in an airtight container.

The buckwheat and quinoa granola can yield six servings.

7. **Cherry Quinoa Porridge**

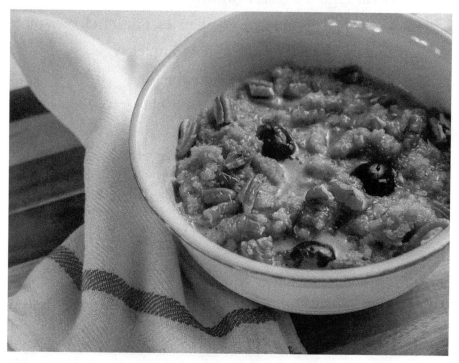

Serves 2; Directions time - 2 minutes

Ingredients:

- Water (1 cup)
- Dry quinoa (1 cup)
- Dried unsweetened cherries (1 cup)
- Vanilla extract (1/2 tsp)
- Ground cinnamon (¼ tsp)
- Honey (¼ tsp), optional

Directions:

1. Get a medium-sized saucepan and stir all the ingredients (except honey)

together. Over medium-high heat, bring everything to a boil.

2. Lower the heat, cover the saucepan and simmer. Wait for 15 minutes or until the water is completely absorbed and the quinoa is all tender.

3. If desired, drizzle with some honey before serving.

8. Gingerbread Oatmeal

Serves 1; Directions time – 10 minutes

Ingredients:

- Water (1 cup)
- Old-fashioned oats (½ cup)
- Dried, unsweetened cranberries or cherries (¼ cup)
- Ground ginger (1 tsp)
- Ground cinnamon (½ teaspoon)
- Ground nutmeg (¼ teaspoon)
- Flaxseeds (1 tablespoon)
- Molasses (1 tablespoon)

Directions:

1. Mix the water, oats, cranberries or cherries, ginger, cinnamon, and nutmeg in a small-sized saucepan and heat over medium high settings. Bring the mixture into a boil, then reduce the heat. Simmer for 5 minutes or until such time that the water has been almost completely absorbed.

2. Put the flaxseeds, then cover the saucepan. Let the mixture stand for another 5 minutes.

3. Drizzle the dish with some molasses before serving.

9. <u>Spanish Frittata</u>

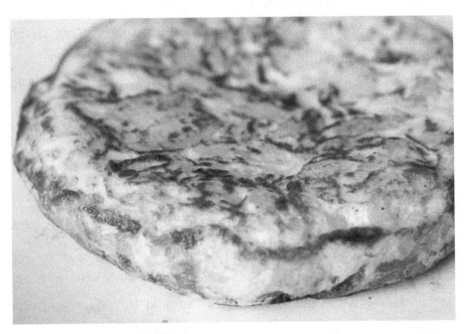

Serves 4 to 6

Ingredients (for the frittata):

- Large organic eggs (1 dozen)
- Coconut milk (½ cup)
- Sea salt (½ tsp, or more to taste)
- Extra-virgin olive oil or coconut oil (2 tbsp)
- Small, finely chopped red onion (1 pc)
- Sautéed mushrooms or vegetable of your choice (½ cup)
- Spinach or arugula (1 cup)

Directions:

1. Pre-heat the oven set at a temperature of 375°F.

2. Whisk the coconut milk and eggs together as you sprinkle two pinches of salt; then set aside.

3. Get a pan and heat coconut oil at medium-high setting. Sauté onions for about 3 minutes or until translucent.

4. Add the mushrooms or vegetables of your choice and sauté until they soften.

5. Put the spinach in and fold into the vegetable mixture just until they wilt. Remove the veggies from the pan and set aside.

6. Adjust the heat to low setting, while adding just a bit more coconut oil, if necessary. With the same skillet, place the eggs while shaking to evenly distribute the mixture.

7. Set the heat to medium-low then cook for about 5 more minutes. Use a spatula to gather the eggs at the edges and mix them with the rest of the ingredients at the center. Do this until there are no more runny edges. Arrange the veggie mix evenly over the top.

8. Move the dish to the oven and resume cooking for 5 more minutes or until it is set and browned slightly.

9. Turn off the heat and take the dish out of the oven; be wary of the hot handle as you do this so it is best to wear oven mitts first.

10. Finish everything off by sliding the slightly cooked frittata onto a big serving plate.

11. Place a plate on top of the pan. Hold together the pan and the plate then invert them in a way that the frittata falls on the plate.

12. Slide it back to the pan so that the slightly cooked side is on top.

13. Put the dish back into the oven and cook for another 3 or 4 minutes. Serve with a simple siding of salad with citrus vinaigrette.

10. <u>**Orange Apple Breakfast Shake**</u>

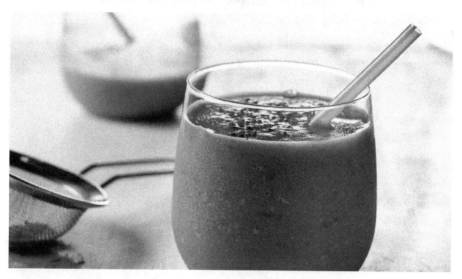

Serves 1; Directions time – 10 minutes

Ingredients

- Almonds (2 tbsp.)
- Apple slices (1/2 cup)
- Orange sections (1/2 cup)
- 2% milk (1 cup)
- Zone Protein Powder (14g)

Directions:

1. Place all ingredients together in the blender. Mix until everything is wellincorporated

and smooth.

2. Pour the contents of the blender into a tall glass.

3. Serve and enjoy!

11. <u>**Chocolate Cherry Shake**</u>

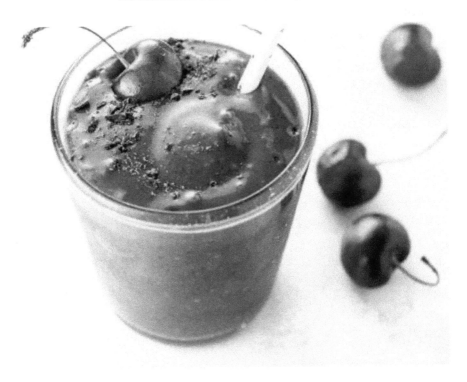

Serves 1

Ingredients:

- Unprocessed, unsweetened cocoa powder (1 tbsp.)
- Frozen dark cherries, pitted (½ cup)
- Coconut, almond or flax milk (1 cup)
- Pure vanilla extract; a few drops of liquid stevia preferably Sweet Leaf Vanilla
- Crème (½ tsp)
- Ice cubes, if desired

Directions:

1. Mix all the ingredients in a blender. Process until everything is smooth.

2. Pour in a tall glass.

3. Serve and enjoy!

12. <u>Oatmeal Spiced Apple Pie</u>

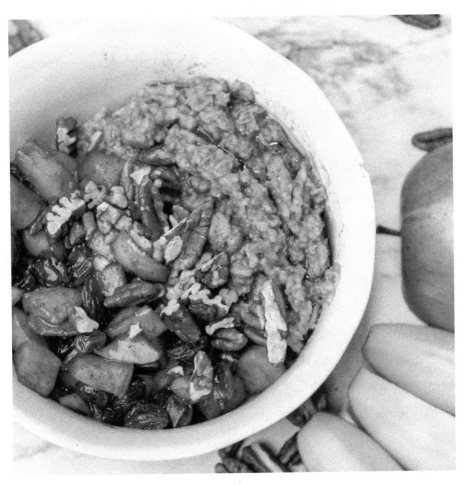

Serves 4; Directions time – 45 minutes

Ingredients:

- Water (3 cups)
- Steel Cut Oats (3/4 cup)
- Pumpkin Spice - Pumpkin Pie Spice (2 tsp)
- Zone Protein Powder (70 grams)
- Applesauce (1 cup)

- Stevia Extract (1 tsp, to taste)
- 16 Pecans or walnuts (16 pcs – halves)

Directions:

1. Boil the water before stirring in the pumpkin pie spice and steel-cut oats.

Cook for about 5 minutes then reduce the heat. Simmer for half an hour.

Let the dish col off before stirring in the protein powder. (This can be prepared the previous evening, refrigerate, and then just heat in the microwave oven the following morning.) Add the rest of the ingredients once you are about to eat.

2. If prepared the previous night, take the dish out of the refrigerator and pour into 4 individual bowls.

3. Distribute the rest of the ingredients among the 4 bowls and warm up in the microwave oven for 2 ½ minutes under high temperature setting.

4. Stir while halfway through.

13. <u>Eggs and Fruit Salad</u>

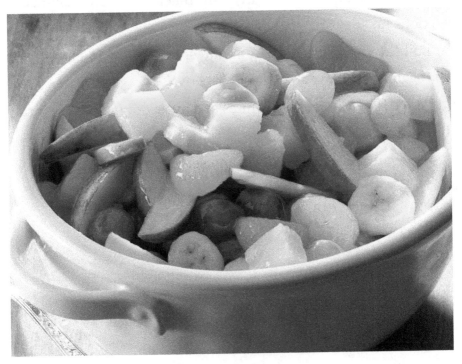

Serves 1; Directions time – 20 minutes

Ingredients:

- Strawberries, sliced (1/2 cup)
- Mandarin orange sections, unsweetened or fresh (1/2 cup)
- Blueberries (1/2 cup)
- Egg whites (6 hardboiled eggs, discard yolks)
- Avocado (1/2 cup)
- Salsa (3 tbsp.)

Directions:

1. Prepare the fruit salad in a medium-sized bowl. Slice strawberries, and then gently stir blueberries and mandarin sections in.

2. Boil the eggs for about 10 minutes, then allow to cool. Halve the eggs and remove the yolks.

3. Dice the hardboiled egg whites and avocado; mix in a separate bowl. Stir the salsa in.

4. Put some fruit salad sidings, and serve.

14. Ham & Onion Frittata w/ Fruit Salad

Serves 4; Directions time – 30 minutes

Ingredients:

- Cooking spray (olive oil)
- Onion, chopped (1 pc)
- Canadian bacon, cut in bite sized pieces (4 oz)
- Egg whites (2 cups)
- Olive oil (1 tbsp.)
- 1% milk (1/4 cup)
- Dried dill (1 tbsp or 3 tbsp if fresh)
- Salt and pepper, to taste
- Mozzarella cheese, shredded (3/4 cup)
- Parmesan cheese, grated (1/4 cup)
- Blueberries (1 cup, divided)
- Freshly squeezed lemon juice (3 tbsp)
- Vanilla 1 1/2 tsps
- Agave nectar (1 ½ tbsp.)
- Peach, sliced (1 pc)
- Pear, sliced (1pc)
- Strawberries, sliced (1 ½ cups)

Directions:

1. Spray olive oil in a large ovenproof skillet. Saute the ham and onion until
the onion is cooked and golden. Set them aside.

2. Pre-heat the oven for broiling.

3. Whisk together the egg whites, milk, olive oil, dill, and salt & pepper in a medium-sized bowl. Add the cheeses into the mix.

4. Spread the cooled ham and onion evenly at the bottom of the skillet. Top with the egg mixture. Cook under medium heat setting until the bottom settles.

5. Put the skillet under broiler, and then cook some more until the eggs are set and the top is golden brown. Remove the skillet from the oven and set it aside and allow to cool off.

6. Take ¼ cup of blueberries and mix with vanilla, agave nectar, and lemon juice in a small-sized bowl. Set the mixture aside.

7. Mix the sliced fruits and blueberries in a large-sized bowl. Pour the sauce mixture over the fruits and mix everything up.

8. Serve and enjoy with the frittata.

15. <u>Grapefruit Breakfast</u>

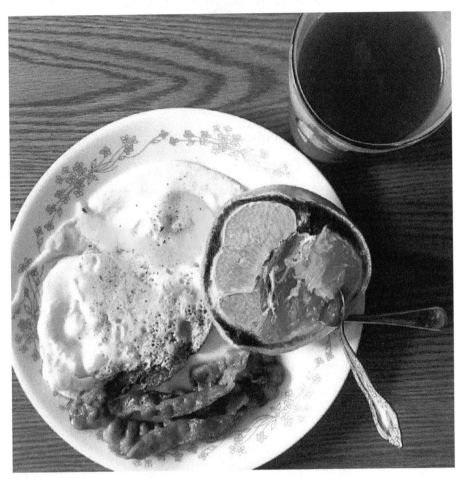

Serves 1; Directions time – 5 minutes

Ingredients:

- Canadian bacon (2 slices)
- Grapefruit (1 pc)
- 0%-fat Greek yogurt (1/2 cup)
- Blueberries (1/3 cup)
- Sliced almonds (3 1/2 tbsp.)

Directions:

1. Get the slices of Canadian bacon and cut into smaller pieces. Place in the microwave oven to warm.

2. Cut the grapefruit into two, then slice each section into smaller pieces.
Place the pieces in a bowl. Stir the Canadian bacon in.

3. Next, get another bowl and mix the almonds and blueberries with yogurt.

4. Combine the contents of the two bowls and mix well.

5. Serve and enjoy!

16. <u>Vanilla Cherry Quinoa</u>

Directions Time: 20 Minutes

Serves: 2

Ingredients:

- 1.5 cup water
- ¾ cup dry Quinoa
- ¾ cup unsweetened, dried cherries
- 2 tsp Vanilla Extract
- 1 – 2 pinch ground Cinnamon

Directions:

1. Stir in the ingredients (except honey) into a medium sized sauce pan over a medium-high flame and bring to a boil.

2. Once the mix boils, reduce the heat, cover the pan and allow the contents to simmer for about 15 minutes or until the water has been absorbed completely and the quinoa is soft.

3. Serve into bowls and drizzle with honey (if required).

17. <u>Raspberry Green Tea Power Smoothie</u>

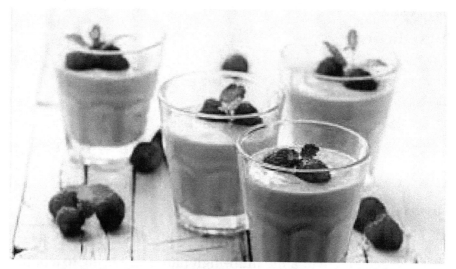

Directions Time: 10 Minutes

Serves: 2

Ingredients

- 2 cups Green Tea – chilled
- 1 large cup Raspberries, frozen
- 1 small Banana
- 2 scoops Protein powder
- 2 tsp Honey

Directions:

1. Add all the ingredients to a blender, blitz until you get a smooth puree.
2. Pour into tall glasses and enjoy!

18.   <u>Sweet Spiced Oats</u>

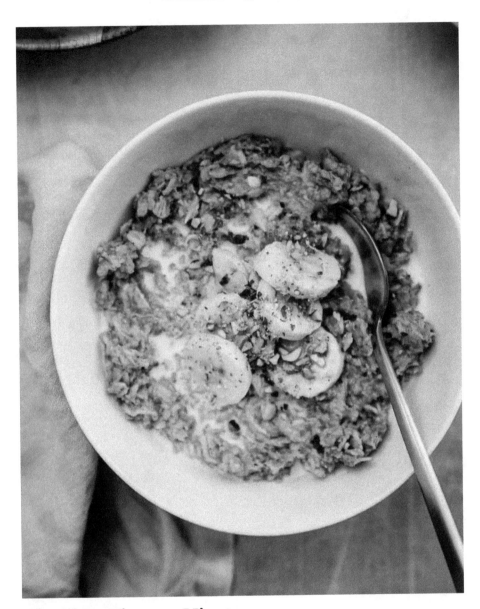

Directions Time: 10 Minutes

Serves: 2

Ingredients

- 2 cups Water
- 1 cup Oats
- ½ cup dried Cranberries / Cherries
- 1 tsp Cinnamon powder
- 1 tsp Nutmeg powder
- 2 tbsp. Molasses
- 2 tbsp. Flaxseeds

Directions:

1. In a small saucepan, combine all ingredients except the flaxseed and molasses and bring to a boil over a medium-high heat.
2. Once the mixture boils, reduce the heat, cover and allow it to simmer for about 5 minutes until all the water is absorbed.
3. Add flaxseeds and cover for about 5 minutes off the heat.
4. Drizzle with molasses and serve.

19. <u>Sweet and Savoury Breakfast Muffins</u>

Directions Time: 30 minutes

Serves: 4 – 6

Ingredients:

- 3 cups All-Purpose Flour
- 1 cup Sugar
- 2 tsp Baking Powder
- 1 pinch of Salt
- 1.5 tsp Cinnamon powder
- 1.5 tsp Ginger – ground.
- 1 cup Almond milk (unsweetened)
- 2 Apples – shredded
- ¾ cup mashed, ripe Banana
- 1.5 tbsp. Apple Cider vinegar
- ¾ cup Crystallized ginger – finely chopped

Directions:

1. Preheat the oven to 400°F. Lightly grease a muffin pan or use liners (12 cup pan should suffice).

2. Whisk together the flour, sugar, baking powder, salt and spices in a medium bowl to make the flour mix.

3. In another bowl, mix the milk, banana, apples, apple cider vinegar and crystallized ginger. To this, add the flour mixture until you get a consistent batter.

4. Pour the batter into the muffin pan/liners till the cups are about 2/3 full.

5. Bake the muffins at 400°F for about 15-20 minutes.

20. <u>Quinoa Buckwheat Flapjacks</u>

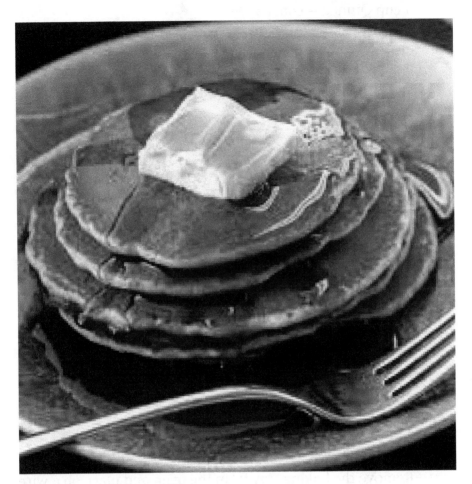

Directions Time: 1 Hour

Serves: 3 – 4

Ingredients

- 4 Tbsp. Honey
- 4 Tbsp. cold pressed Coconut Oil
- 2 tsp Vanilla Extract
- ¼ tsp Cinnamon powder

- ¼ tsp Ginger – ground
- 1 cup Quinoa – cooked
- 1 cup Buckwheat groats
- 1 cup Oats
- 1 cup dried Cranberries

Directions:

1. Preheat the oven to 325°F.
2. Grease a baking pan or line with a parchment sheet and put aside.
3. Add the coconut oil, honey, vanilla, cinnamon and ginger in a small bowl and mix well.
4. In a large bowl, combine together the Buckwheat, Cranberries, Quinoa and Oats.
5. Add the mixture from the small bowl and stir vigorously to combine. Spread this mixture on to the baking pan in an even, uniform layer.
6. Place the baking tray in the oven and bake at 325°F for about 45 minutes until the grains start to brown.
7. Remove the baking tray from the oven and place on a wire rack to cool.
8. Cut into bite sized pieces and store in an airtight container.

21. <u>Oriental Baked Omelettes</u>

Directions Time: 1 hour

SERVES: 6

Ingredients

- 500 gm sliced Button Mushrooms
- 2 medium Onions, chopped
- 2 tbsp. Garlic, finely chopped
- 500 gm Fresh Spinach leaves, roughly chopped.
- ½ cup Water
- 6 Egg Whites
- 4 large Eggs
- 5 oz. Tofu
- 1 – 2 pinch Turmeric powder
- Salt and Pepper to taste.

Directions:

1. Preheat the oven to 350°F. Sauté the mushrooms in a lightly greased oven-proof skillet or pan until the mushrooms are golden brown. To this, add the onions and cook till they are soft. Add the chopped garlic to this and cook for another 20 seconds.

2. Add the spinach and water, and cook with the lid on for about 2 minutes until the spinach wilts. Remove the lid and cook further until the water has evaporated.

3. In a blender, add the tofu, egg whites and egg with the turmeric powder, salt and pepper and blend till smooth. Pour this egg mixture gently over the spinach and

4. mushrooms.

5. Transfer the pan to the oven and bake for about 20 minutes at 350°F so that the eggs are set in the center.

6. Remove the pan from the oven and invert over a plate and allow to cool.

7. Cut the omelette into wedges and serve!

22. <u>Nutty Protein Oats</u>

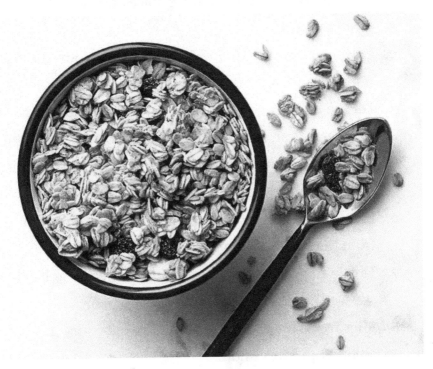

Directions Time: 1 hour

Serves: 3 – 4

Ingredients

- 4 cups Water
- 1 cup Steel Cut Oats
- 3 tsp Pumpkin Pie Spice
- 10 scoops Protein powder
- 1.5 cup Apple Sauce
- 1 tsp Honey/Agave/Stevia extract
- 15 – 20 Pecans or Walnuts

Directions:

1. In a saucepan, bring the water to a boil and stir in the steel cut oats with the pumpkin pie spice and allow this to cook for 5 minutes.

2. Lower the heat and allow this to simmer for another 30 minutes and take off the flame.

3. Let the mixture cool and then stir in the protein powder.

4. This recipe can be prepared the night before, stored in the fridge and warmed up in the microwave in the morning.

5. Add the rest of the ingredients when you are ready to eat!

6. If this is prepared the night before, then remove the oats from the fridge and serve in individual bowls.

7. Divide the remaining ingredients between the bowls and stir well.

8. Microwave for about 2 minutes on high, stirring every 30 seconds and serve hot!

23. <u>Baked Cheesy Eggs</u>

Directions Time: 1 hour

Serves: 2

Ingredients

- 8 Roma Tomatoes, peeled and chopped in to small pieces
- 2 tbsp. Olive Oil
- 2 tbsp. Vegetable stock
- 1 medium Onion – finely chopped
- 100 gm Ham – roughly chopped
- 150gm Spinach – chopped
- 5 large Egg Whites
- ¼ cup Cream Cheese (can substitute with dairy free cheese too)
- ¼ small cup fresh Chives – chopped
- 4 tbsp. Almond milk – unsweetened

Directions:

1. Preheat the oven to 350°F. Coat the inner surface of two oven-safe bowls with olive oil or any other organic virgin oil.
2. In a separate bowl, toss together the tomatoes and salt.
3. Spoon this content between the two greased bowls, and set them aside. In another large skillet, add oil and then onions.
4. Once the onions are translucent, add vegetable stock and cook over a medium heat, stirring

5. occasionally for 4 minutes. Add the chopped ham and cook for another minute more, and remove the pan from the heat. Add the spinach and toss lightly in the ham and onion mixture to wilt the leaves lightly and then add this to the two bowls with the tomatoes.

6. In another bowl, whisk the egg whites, cream cheese, chopped chives and almond milk.

7. Add this to the bowls having the tomato mixture.

8. Place the bowls on a baking tray or pan that is large enough to hold the both of them, and place the tray on the middle rack in the oven.

9. Pour boiling water carefully onto the pan so that the bowls are submerged about half way.

10. Bake them for about 30 minutes.

11. Once done, remove the bowls carefully from the tray and season with salt and pepper, serve hot.

12. You can optionally garnish the dish with orange slices for an extra burst of flavor.

24. <u>Berry Nut Burst</u>

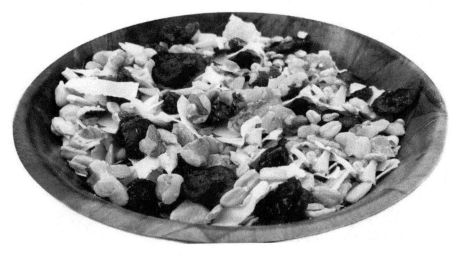

Directions Time: 5 Minutes

Serves: 2

Ingredients

- 2 cups Strawberries
- 1.5 cup Blueberries
- 1.4 cup Walnuts and Pecans (roughly chopped)
- 2 cups fat-free Greek Yogurt

Directions:

1. Mix the berries and nuts into the yogurt, scoop into bowls.
2. Garnish with a mint leaf and serve!

25. <u>Provolone Egg White Omelette</u>

Directions Time: 15 Minutes

Serves: 2

Ingredients

- 2 tbsp. Olive oil
- ½ cup Onions – diced
- ½ cup Green Peppers – diced
- ½ cup Garbanzo Beans – canned
- 1 cup Egg whites
- 1 cup Salsa
- 2 slices low fat Provolone Cheese
- ½ cup Mandarin – sliced, in water

Seasoning -

- Basil
- Oregano
- Salt & Pepper

Directions:

1. In a pan, add 2 tbsp. of olive oil and heat. Add the peppers and onions until they have softened. Drain the Garbanzo beans, rinse thoroughly and slightly mash
2. them.
3. Add the beans to the pan and sauté gently.
4. In a bowl, beat the egg whites till they are lightly foamy. Add the spices to this, and whisk lightly once again.

5. Gently pour the egg whites over the cooking beans, onions and peppers making sure you cover the whole pan.

6. Add the cheese, cover and let the eggs cook on a low medium heat until the cheese is melted and the eggs are cooked.

7. Serve onto a plate, fold in half and top with the salsa.

8. You can add the mandarin slices as a garnish.

26. **Chicken and Tomato Omelette**

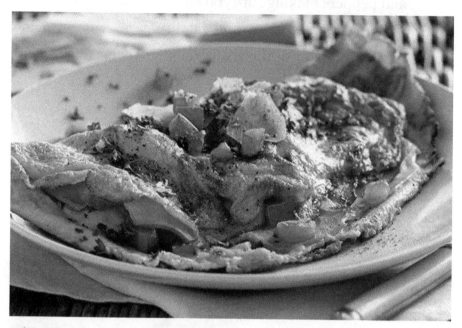

Directions Time: 30 Minutes

Serves: 4

Ingredients

- 500 gm Broccoli
- 1.5 cup sun dried Tomatoes - finely chopped
- 1.5 cup Egg whites
- 2/3 cup low fat milk
- 2/3 cup Cottage Cheese – low fat
- 3 tbsp. Olive Oil
- 4 – 5 tbsp. Pesto (any store bought recipe will do)
- Salt and Pepper
- 5 oz. roasted/grilled/boiled Chicken breast

- 4 cloves Garlic – finely minced
- 4 tsp Capers
- 4 Oranges

Directions:

1. Cover a medium skillet with cooking oil spray, and add the broccoli to it.
2. Add about 2/3 cup water to it and cover.
3. Cook the broccoli for about 5 – 8 minutes, remove from the heat and drain thoroughly.
4. In a large bowl, mix together the egg whites, cottage cheese, pesto, salt, pepper and olive oil, whisking briskly.
5. Add chicken, garlic and capers sun dried tomatoes to this and pour the mixture gently into a clean skillet.
6. Cover and let this cook on a medium heat till one side is set.
7. Carefully turn this over, and allow the eggs to finish cooking.

27. <u>Lean Eating Oatmeal</u>

Serves: 4 servings

Ingredients

Maple syrup to taste

- ¼ teaspoon ground cardamom
- 1/8 teaspoon ground nutmeg
- ¼ teaspoon ground allspice
- ¼ teaspoon ground ginger
- 1 teaspoon ground coriander
- 1½ tablespoons ground cinnamon
- 1 cup steel cut oats
- 4 cups water

Directions

1. Cook the oats in accordance with the package directions making sure to include the

spices when you add the oats to the water.

2. Add maple syrup to taste.

28. Buckwheat and Ginger Granola

Serves: 1 serving

Ingredients

- A piece of ginger (20g)
- 4 tablespoons of raw cacao powder
- 6 tablespoons of coconut oil
- 1 cup apple puree
- 1½ cups pitted dates
- 1 cup pumpkin seeds
- 1 cup sunflower seeds
- 1 cup buckwheat
- 2 cups of oats

Directions

1. Pre-heat your oven to 180°c.

2. Place the buckwheat, oats, and seeds in a large mixing bowl and stir well.

3. In a saucepan, add the dates, apple puree, and coconut oil and allow the mixture to simmer for 5 minutes, or until the dates are soft and nice.

4. As the dates cook, peel the ginger and grate it onto a plate. Once it is grated, mix the ginger into the date pan.

5. Once the dates are soft, place the contents of your pan in a blender together with the raw cacao powder and blend until the mixture is smooth. Pour the mixture over the buckwheat, seed mix, and oat, and stir well until you coat everything.

6. Use coconut oil to grease one large baking tray. Spread the granola on the tray, place them in the oven, and bake for about 45 minutes, stirring everything well after every 15 minutes to keep the granola from burning.

7. Once crispy, take the granola out of the oven and allow it to cool. For storage, put in an airtight container.

29. <u>**Chia Lemon Quinoa**</u>

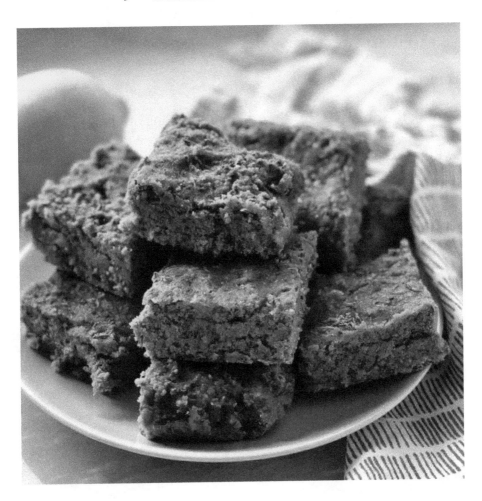

Serves: 6 servings

Ingredients

- 1 ½ cups almond milk
- 1 cup quinoa
- ¼ teaspoon sea salt
- 1 tablespoon chia seeds

- 3 tablespoons slivered almonds
- 4 ½ tablespoons pure maple syrup
- Pinch of fresh lemon zest

Directions

1. Cook the quinoa according to the directions on the package.

2. Remove from the heat then put aside for around five minutes then fluff using a fork and add, maple syrup, almond milk, chia seeds, almonds, lemon zest and sea salt then combine well and serve warm.

30. <u>Spicy Green Bean 'Fries'</u>

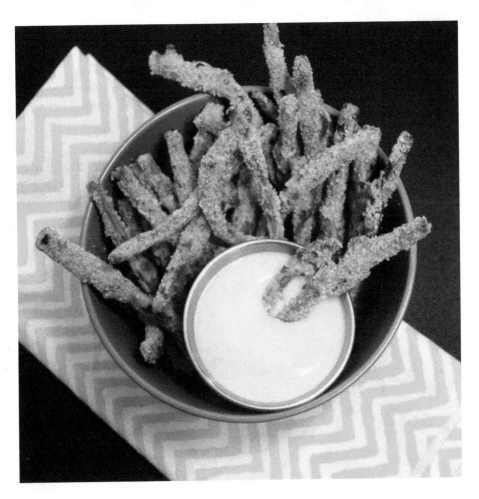

Serves: 2 servings

Ingredients

- A dash of chili powder
- 3 cups of cold water
- 3 cups of hot water
- 2 cups green beans

- Sea salt and pepper to taste

Directions

1. Wash and trim the green beans.

2. Boil water in a small saucepan, and add a pinch of salt. Add the beans and blanch for about 2 minutes.

3. Using tongs, remove all the beans and place them in cold water to stop the cooking process.

4. Dry the beans, and season with chili, pepper, and salt.

31. <u>Chocolate Cupcakes With Sweet Potato Frosting</u>

Serves: 12 servings

Ingredients

Cupcake

- ½ cup baking soda
- 1 teaspoon baking powder
- ½ cup walnuts
- ¾ cup mineral water
- ½ cup cacao powder
- ½ cup 100% pure maple syrup
- ½ cup unsweetened dried coconut
- 1 apple, cored and cut into 1/8ths
- ½ cup buckwheat groats
- ½ cup millet

Frosting

- 1/8 cinnamon
- ½ tablespoon of 100% pure maple syrup
- ¼ cup walnuts
- 3 dates, pitted and simmered in water for 5 minutes.
- ½ cup cooked sweet potato

Directions

1. Soak the millet and buckwheat for a day.

2. Preheat your oven to 350°F.

3. Drain and rinse the grains. Place them in a blender along with walnuts, mineral water, cacao powder, maple syrup, coconut, and the apple. Blend until smooth.

4. Pour the batter into a mixing bowl and add baking soda and powder. Whisk until everything mixes.

5. Line your muffin tin with liners and fill each one with batter.

6. Bake the cupcakes for 35 minutes.

7. While the baking occurs, place the cooked sweet potato, cinnamon, maple syrup, dates and walnut in a blender and blend until creamy and smooth.

8. After baking and cooling, spread a generous amount of frosting on each cupcake and serve.

32. <u>Coconut Cake Protein Balls</u>

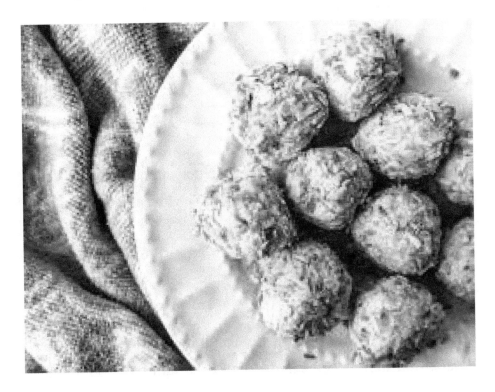

Serves: 18 servings

Ingredients

- 1/3 cup unsweetened shredded coconut
- ¼ cup pecans
- ¼ cup walnuts
- 4 tablespoons unsweetened applesauce
- 1/8 teaspoon ground ginger
- ¼ teaspoon nutmeg
- ½ teaspoon cinnamon

- 1 scoop protein powder
- 1 carrot, shredded
- 6 pitted dates
- ¾ cup rolled oats
- 2 cups cashews

Directions

1. Mix the cashews, the spices, protein powder, applesauce, dates, and oats in a blender and blend until you get a chunky dough.

2. Add the shredded carrots, walnuts, and the pecans to the blender and mix until uniformly mixed.

3. Add the shredded coconut to a separate bowl.

4. Take a spoonful of dough and roll it into individual bite-sized balls. Roll then in the shredded coconut and place on a baking dish or plate.

5. Place the balls in the refrigerator for about 45 minute before you serve.

33. <u>Oatmeal and Cinnamon with Dried Cranberries</u>

SERVES 2 / PREP TIME 5 MINUTES / COOK TIME 8 MINUTES

- 1 Cup Water
- 1 Cup Almond Milk
- Pinch Sea Salt
- 1 Cup Old-Fas Hioned Oats
- ½ Cup Dried Cranberries
- 1 Teas Poon Ground Cinnamon

Directions:

1. In a medium saucepan over high heat, bring the water, almond milk, and salt to a boil.
2. Stir in the oats, cranberries, and cinnamon. Reduce the heat to medium and cook for 5 minutes, stirring occasionally.
3. Remove the oatmeal from the heat. Cover the pot and let it stand for 3 minutes. Stir before serving.

34. **Baked oatmeal**

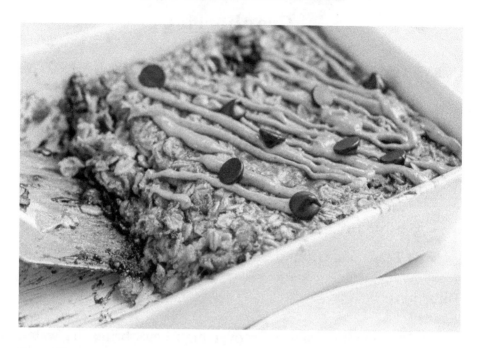

Ingredients

- 2 cups/7 oz/200 g rolled oats
- 1/2 cup/2 oz/60 g walnut pieces, toasted and chopped
- 1/3 cup/2 oz/60 g natural cane sugar or maple syrup, plus more for
- serving
- 1 teaspoon aluminum-free baking powder
- 1 1/2 teaspoons ground cinnamon
- Scant 1/2 teaspoon fine-grain sea salt
- 2 cups/475 ml milk
- 1 large egg

- 3 tablespoons unsalted butter, melted and cooled slightly
- 2 teaspoons pure vanilla extract
- 2 ripe bananas, cut into 1/2-inch/1 cm pieces
- 1 1/2 cups/6.5 oz/185 g huckleberries, blueberries, or mixed berries

Directions

1. Preheat the oven to 375°F/190°C with a rack in the top third of the oven.

Generously butter the inside of an 8-inch/20cm square baking dish.

2. In a bowl, mix together the oats, half the walnuts, the sugar, if using, the

baking powder, cinnamon, and salt.

3. In another bowl, whisk together the maple syrup, if using, the milk, egg,

half of the butter, and the vanilla.

4. Arrange the bananas in a single layer in the bottom of the prepared

baking dish.

5. Sprinkle two-thirds of the berries over the top.

6. Cover the fruit with the oat mixture.

7. Slowly drizzle the milk mixture over the oats. Gently give the baking

dish a couple thwacks on the countertop to make sure the milk moves

through the oats. Scatter the remaining berries and remaining walnuts

across the top.

8. Bake for 35 to 45 minutes, until the top is nicely golden and the oat

mixture has set.

9. Remove from the oven and let cool for a few minutes.

10. Drizzle the remaining melted butter on the top and serve.

11. Sprinkle with a bit more sugar or drizzle with maple syrup if you want it

a bit sweeter.

35. **Breakfast casserole**

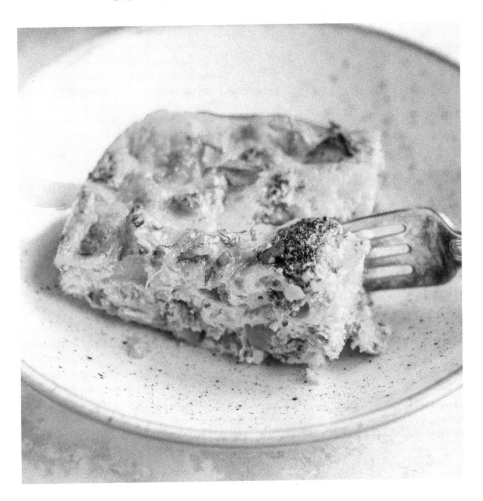

Ingredients

- 6 slices soft hearty white bread
- One 8-ounce package shredded triple cheddar cheese
- 8 large eggs
- 2 cups whole milk
- 1 teaspoon dry mustard

- ¼ teaspoon salt
- ½ teaspoon seasoned pepper

Directions

1. Preheat the oven to 350 degrees F. Spray a 13-by 9-inch baking sheet with nonstick cooking spray.

2. In a large skillet, cook the sausage over medium heat, stirring frequently,until brown and crumbly, about 10 minutes; drain well on paper

3. Cut and discard the crust of the bread. Cut the slices in half, and arrange

in a single layer in the prepared baking dish, cutting pieces to fit as necessary to cover the bottom of the dish. Sprinkle with the sausage and cheese.

4. In a large bowl, whisk together the eggs, milk, mustard, seasoned and pepper; carefully pour the mixture over the cheese.

5. Bake casserole until set and golden, about 40 minutes.

6. Let stand for 10 minutes before serving .

36. __Pumpkin pancakes__

Ingredients

- 1 1⁄4 cups all-purpose flour
- 2 tablespoons sugar
- 2 teaspoons baking powder
- 1⁄2 teaspoon cinnamon
- 1⁄2 teaspoon ginger
- 1⁄2 teaspoon nutmeg
- 1⁄2 teaspoon salt
- 1 pinch clove
- 1 cup 1% low-fat milk (can be any kind)
- 6 tablespoons canned pumpkin puree
- 2 tablespoons melted butter
- 1 egg

Directions

1. Whisk flour, sugar, baking powder, spices and salt in a bowl.

2. In a separate bowl whisk together milk, pumpkin, melted butter, and egg.

3. Fold mixture into dry ingredients.

4. Spray or grease a skillet and heat over medium heat: pour in 1/4 cup

batter for each pancake.

5. Cook pancakes about 3 minutes per side. Serve with butter and syrup.

6. Makes about six 6-inch pancakes.

37. <u>Cornflakes, Low-Fat Milk and berries</u>

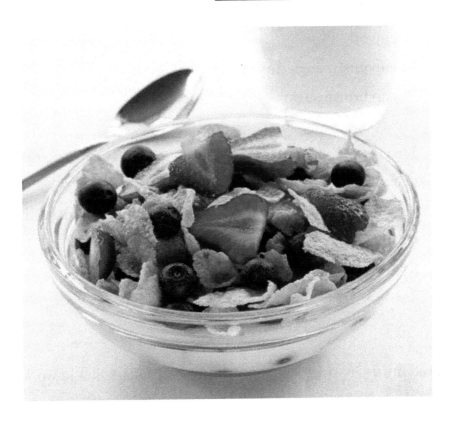

Ingredients

- 2 cups cornflakes
- 1 cup 1% low-fat milk
- 1 cup berries, fresh or frozen, thawed

Directions

1. Place cornflakes in a small bowl. Top with milk and berries.

38. <u>Low Cook Oatmeal</u>

ingredients

- ¼ cup oil
- ¼ cup unsweetened applesauce
- ¾ cup brown sugar
- 1 teaspoon cinnamon
- 1 teaspoon salt
- 2 large eggs
- 1-1/2 cups skim milk (I used vanilla coconut milk beverage)
- 3 cups uncooked oatmeal, rolled or quick oats
- 2 teaspoons baking powder

Directions

1. I used my 2-Quart Crockpot for this but a 3-Quart should work too.

2. Coat your slow cooker with nonstick cooking spray.

3. In a large bowl whisk together the oil, applesauce, brown sugar, salt, and

eggs until well blended and creamy. Whisk in the milk.

4. Add the oats and baking powder and stir until well mixed.

5. Pour into your greased slow cooker.

6. Cover and cook on LOW for 3 to 5 hours, until the edges are golden brown

and the center is set. (Mine was done in 4 hours.)

7. Serve hot or let it stand in the slow cooker for up to an hour and then cut it into pieces for serving.

39. <u>Banana Cream Pie</u>

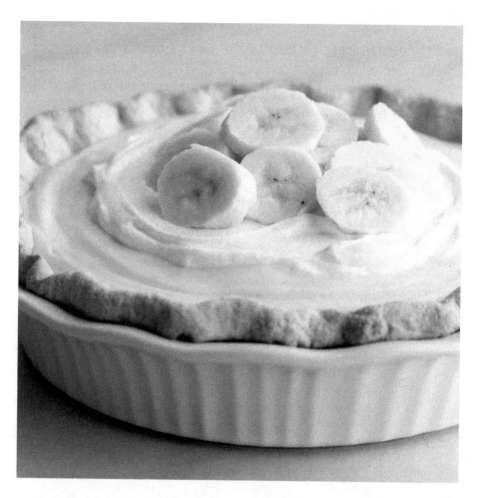

Ingredients

- ½ cup plain nonfat Greek yogurt
- ½ banana thinly sliced, (Make sure it's ripe with some spots since it will be
- sweeter.)
- 1 teaspoon wheat germ

- ¼ teaspoon vanilla extract
- Drizzle of honey

Directions

1. In a small bowl, stir together the yogurt, sliced bananas, vanilla, and wheat germ. Drizzle with honey.

40. **Egg Salad**

Ingredients

- 6 hard boiled eggs, peeled and chopped
- 2 tablespoons light Hellman's mayonnaise
- 3 tablespoons plain nonfat Greek yogurt
- 2 teaspoons mustard
- ¼ teaspoon salt
- ¼ teaspoon ground black pepper

Optional Egg Salad Additions

- ¼ cup finely chopped celery
- 2 tablespoons, minced red onion or green onion (scallion)
- 2 teaspoons lemon juice
- 1 to 2 tablespoon chopped fresh parsley
- 1 to 2 tablespoons chopped fresh dill

Directions

1. In a medium bowl mix all ingredients, and any optional ingredients from

the list below, until well blended.

41. **Walnut Oatmeal and Yogurt**

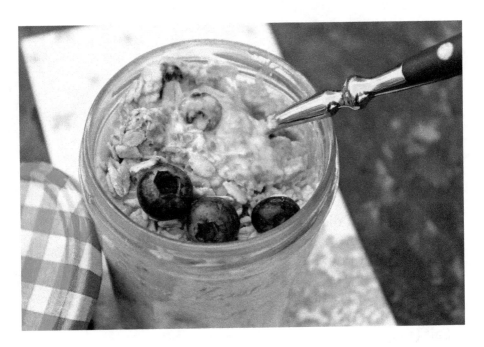

Ingredients

- 1 cup Oatmeal, cooked
- 1 tablespoon Chopped Walnuts
- 4 tablespoons Plain Greek Yogurt
- ½ cup Blueberries

Directions

1. Top Oatmeal with walnuts.

2. Top yogurt with blueberries

42. <u>Veggie Egg Muffins</u>

Serves: 8

Time required for proper Directions: 20 minutes

Suggested cooking time: 30 minutes

Total required: 50 minutes

What to Use

- Onion (1 small, diced)

- Mushrooms (4 medium, sliced)

- Powdered garlic (2 tsp.)

- Salt (1 tsp.)

- Provolone cheese (.25 c shredded)

- Eggs (8)

- Milk (.25 c)

- Broccoli (2 c cut or torn into small florets)

- Bell pepper (1 c chopped)

Directions

1. Ensure your oven is heated to 350F.
2. Grease the muffin pan, and fill with vegetables.
3. In a large bowl, add the eggs, garlic powder & salt.

4. Fill each c.75of the way with the egg mixture then top with a pinch of cheese.

5. Bake approximately 25 to 30 minutes or until puffy and golden brown.

43. <u>Sweet Potato Breakfast Burrito</u>

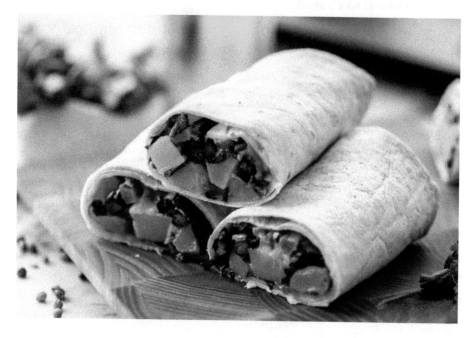

Serves: 1

Time required for proper Directions: 25 minutes

Suggested cooking time: 10 minutes

Total required: 35 minutes

What to Use

- Coconut oil (4 tsp.)

- Cheddar cheese (2 oz. shredded)

- Baby spinach (4 c packed, roughly chopped)

- Sweet potatoes (2 small peeled and diced)

- Yellow onions (2 small, chopped)

- Tricolor bell peppers (1.5 c frozen, sliced, thawed)

- 10-inch whole wheat tortillas (8)

- Chili powder (2 tsp.)

- Eggs (4 large beaten)

- Egg whites (4 large, beaten)

Directions

1. Place your skillet on the stove over a burner turned to medium heat.

2. Sauté potato, onion and bell peppers for approximately 7 minutes.

3. Toss in chili powder, spinach, and sauté for another 2 minutes. Increase the heat slightly to high/medium. Mix in eggs and egg whites.

4. Cook for 3 minutes, continuing to stir until eggs are cooked completely and not runny.

5. Remove from heat and cool for 10 minutes. Cut 8 16-inch pieces of aluminum foil. Place 1 tortilla on top of each piece.

6. Put an equal portion of the egg mixture in the middle of each tortilla. Sprinkle cheese on top.

7. Fold two sides in first, and then roll forward from the top of the burrito. Make sure the foil is wrapped tightly around

the burrito, but not inside the roll, if you will be microwaving it to reheat.

8. Place burritos into a large plastic bag in the fridge. There are two ways to reheat.

9. You can either bake the burrito on a cookie sheet in a 400-degree oven for 35 minutes or cook in the microwave for 2 minutes.

10. Transfer the burrito to a paper

11. bag with a pair of tongs, and you can bring it with you on the run.

44. __Porridge__

Serves: 1

Time required for proper Directions: 5 minutes

Suggested cooking time: 5 minutes

Total required: 10 minutes

What to Use

- Salt (1 pinch)

- Coconut cream (4 T)

- Psyllium husk powder (1 pinch ground)

- Coconut flour (1 T)

- Egg (1)

- Coconut oil (1 oz.)

Directions

1. Place everything together in a small pan before placing the pan on the stove on top of a burner set to low heat.

2. Stir the results continuously to encourage porridge to thicken. Continue stirring until your preferred thickness is reached.

3. A small amount of coconut milk or a few berries (fresh or frozen) can also be added as desired.

45. <u>**Berry Smoothie Bowl**</u>

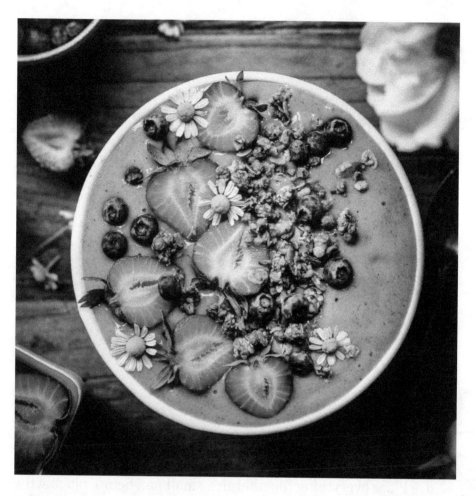

Serves: 1

Time required for proper Directions: 5 minutes

Suggested cooking time: 0 minutes

Total required: 5 minutes

What to Use

- Protein powder (1 scoop)

- Almond milk (2-3 T (can substitute coconut milk))

- Sliced ripe banana (1 that is frozen)

- Organic Frozen mixed berries (1 big c)

- Seeds (Hemp and Chia) (1 T)

- Shreds of coconut (Unsweetened) (1 T)

Directions

1. Blend the berries and ripened banana together.

2. Add the almond milk to the protein powder and blend both until the mixture is blended smoothly. You can top with chia seeds, hemp seeds, or shredded unsweetened coconut if you would like.

3. You can also substitute any non-diary milk if you do not like dairy milk. To

4. take the recipe to another level, you can also substitute a green or white tea as well.

46. <u>Omelet with Mushrooms</u>

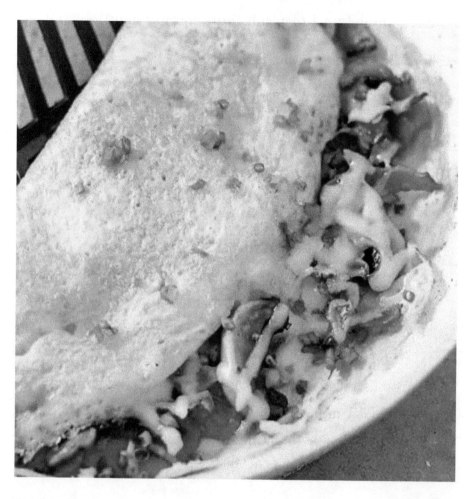

Serves: 1

Time required for proper Directions: 5 minutes

Suggested cooking time: 10 minutes

Total required: 15 minutes

What to Use

- Mushrooms (3 chopped)

- Onion (.25 chopped)

- Sharp cheddar cheese (1 oz. shredded)

- Coconut oil (1 oz. grass fed)

- Pepper (as desired)

- Salt (as desired)

Directions

1. In a mixing bowl, add the eggs and season as desired before whisking well

2. until the eggs become a batter.

3. Add in a majority of the onion, mushroom as well as another pinch of salt to the mixing bowl, and mix well.

4. Add the coconut oil to a frying pan before placing it on top of a burner set to a high/medium heat. Once the coconut oil is completely melted, add in the batter.

5. Once the omelet begins to harden top with the remaining onions and mushrooms before adding the cheese. With the help of a spatula fold the egg on top of itself and continue cooking until it takes on a cooked, golden brown appearance.

47. <u>Scrambled Eggs with Avocado and Bacon</u>

Serves: 4

Preparation: 2 minutes

Cooking time: 10 minutes

Ingredients:

- Pepper (as desired)

- Salt (as desired)

- Bacon (2 oz.)

- Coconut oil (1 tsp.)

- Avocado (.5 peeled)

- Eggs (2)

Directions:

1. Preheat the oven to 350F.
2. In a small pot, place the eggs and add cold water until the eggs are completely covered by roughly 1 inch of water. Add the pot to the stove above a boiler turned to a high/medium heat and let the water boil.
3. After the water has boiled, remove the pot from the stove, let it cool for roughly 10 minutes, and then drain the pot.

4. Fill a large bowl with cold water and dunk the eggs briefly into it to make them easier to peel.

5. Peel and prepare the eggs as preferred before placing them in a bowl, they should be warm, not hot.

6. Split the eggs, remove the yolks, and discard them.

7. In a large bowl, add the eggs, oil, and avocado and mix well before seasoning as desired.

8. Place the bacon on a baking sheet and place the baking sheet in the oven approximately 5 minutes or until done.

9. Once the bacon is no longer hot to the touch, break each piece in half and portion out a half per serving of eggs.

48. <u>Egg Scramble</u>

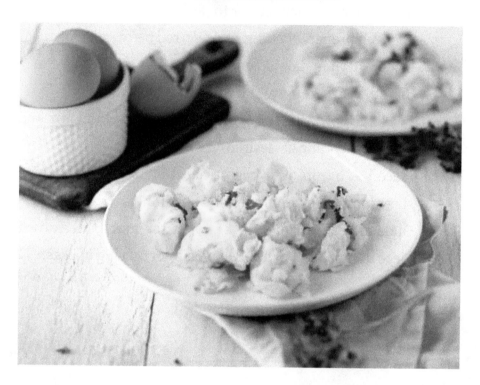

Serves: 2

Preparation Time: 10 minutes

Cooking time: 15 minutes

Ingredients

- Pepper (as desired)

- Salt (as desired)

- Coconut oil (2 T)

- Olives (.5 c pitted)

- Parsley (.5 c chopped)

- Scallions (2)

- Halloumi cheese (4 oz. diced)

- Bacon (5 oz. diced)

- 5 eggs (large)

Directions:

1. Add the oil to a frying pan before placing the pan on the stove on top of a burner set to medium heat. Add in the bacon, scallions, and halloumi and let it all brown.

2. Combine the eggs and parsley in a small bowl and season as desired before whisking.

3. Add the results to the pan before reducing the heat, adding in the olives and stir continuously for 2 additional minutes.

49. **Tabbouleh**

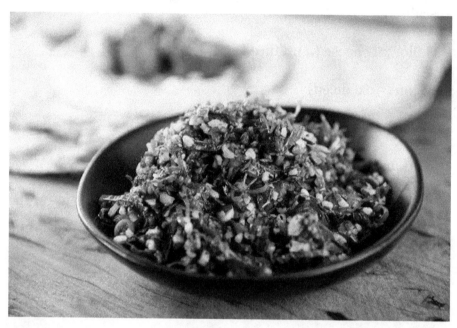

Serves: 4

Preparation Time: 2 hours

Ingredients

- Salt and pepper (as desired)
- Cucumber (1 peeled, seeded, chopped)
- Tomatoes (3 chopped)
- Mint (.25 c chopped)
- Parsley (1 c chopped)
- Green onions (1 c chopped)
- Lemon juice (.3 c)
- Coconut oil (.3 c)
- Water (1.5 c boiling)
- Bulgur (1 c)

Directions:

1. Add the bulgur to the water, cover the pot and let it sit for 60 minutes.

2. Mix in the cucumber, tomatoes, mint, parsley, onions, lemon juice, and oil before seasoning as needed.

3. Add the lid back on and let it sit in the refrigerator for at least 60 minutes before serving.

50. <u>Cherry Coconut Porridge</u>

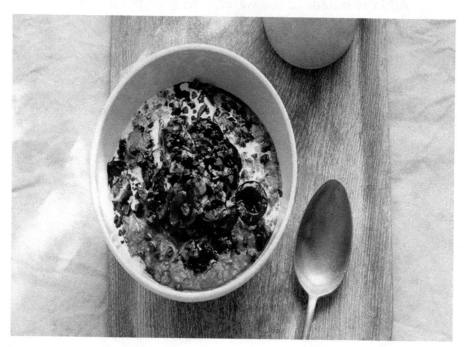

Serves: 1

Preparation Time: 10 minutes

Cooking time: 5 minutes

Total required: 15 minutes

Ingredients:

- Maple syrup (as desired)
- Dark chocolate flakes (as desired)
- Cherries (as desired)
- Coconut shavings (as desired)
- Stevia (1 pinch)
- Cacao (3 T raw)
- Coconut milk (3.5 c)

- Chia seed (4 T)
- Oats (5 c)

Directions:

1. In a saucepan, add the stevia, cacao, coconut milk, chia, and oats together before placing the pan on the stove over a burner turned to medium heat.

2. Let the mixture boil before turning the heat to low and letting everything simmer until the oats are completely cooked.

3. Pour the results into a bowl, add the remaining ingredients as desired and serve hot.

CPSIA information can be obtained
at www.ICGtesting.com
Printed in the USA
LVHW082042220621
690870LV00008B/385